Healing Books

MINERALS

Jon Tillman

Astrolog Publishing House

Pocket Healing Books

Holistic Healing
Dr. Ilona Melman

Aromatherapy
Kevin Hudson

Reiki
Chantal Dupont

Vitamins
Jon Tillman

Bach Flowers
Susan Holden

Herbal Remedies
Dan Wolf

Minerals
Jon Tillman

Color Healing
Barbara White

This publication contains the opinions and ideas of its author. It is intended to provide helpful and informative material on the subject matter covered. It is sold with the understanding that the authors and publisher are not engaged in rendering professional services in the book. If the reader requires personal assistance or advice, a competent professional should be consulted.

The author, book producer, and publisher specifically disclaim any responsibility for any liability, loss or risk, personal or otherwise, which is incurred as a consequence, directly or indirectly, of the use and application of any of the contents of this book.

Introduction

The word "mineral" comes from "mine" - so it means a substance that is extracted from the earth.

The minerals that interest us are elements, which are primary, simple substances that constitute inorganic and organic bodies in nature, as well as in the human body. Minerals are the main components of certain parts of our bodies, such as teeth and bones (calcium), and they play an important role in the electrolytes (the electric transmitters), which are important for the normal functioning of the muscle and nervous systems, as well as for the body's balance or homeostasis.

All the minerals needed by and found in the body are contained in food, and are supplied, under normal circumstances, in the required form and quantity. Food must be the main supplier of the person's minerals, but under certain circumstances, it is necessary to take mineral supplements, mainly because of the absence of their organic form in modern foodstuffs. In addition, supplements are taken when it is necessary to use a mineral as an aid to the body - whether as a solution to a problem that requires a large quantity of the particular mineral, or in order to compensate for a substantial loss of the mineral from the body.

In this book, I will relate to each mineral in

alphabetical order: its role in the body, children's and adults' daily requirements, in which natural sources (foodstuffs) it can be found, food supplements, and toxicity.

It is important to know the links between minerals and vitamins, and these will be indicated during the course of the book, but it must be remembered that the absorption of minerals by the digestive system is linked both to the acid-base balance, and to the combinations of minerals and proteins that require the presence of a protein in the mineral absorption process, and the presence of the appropriate digestive acid.

Minerals that are taken as food supplements must be bound to an amino acid (or some other organic link) in order to enable the mineral to be absorbed effectively.

Minerals that are bound to amino acids are called chealated minerals, and they are absorbed ten times better than minerals that are not bound to amino acids. Another important point is that only 10% of the quantity of non-organic minerals (used in the drug industry) are absorbed, as opposed to natural minerals.

Aluminum

Chemical symbol Al, specific gravity 2.7, atomic weight 26.97 (alumen).

The most widespread metal in the earth's crust, its color resembles silver, it is light and convenient to shape, and for that reason it is used extensively in the disposable utensil industry and kitchen utensil industry (see further on).

For human beings, aluminum is a trace mineral that is also found in foodstuffs and natural food supplements. However, it is liable to cause harm and toxicity in the body.

Large quantities of aluminum have been found in the brains of people who died of Alzheimer's and Parkinson's diseases, and researchers believe that this is directly linked to the diseases (as are other toxicities), as a result of the absorption of the mineral into the tissues.

It is as yet unknown what the role - if any - of aluminum is in the human body, or if it is at all necessary. Nothing is known about a shortage of aluminum - only about excessive amounts. For this reason, **there is no need to take any aluminum**.

Toxicity is aluminum's major problem, and is manifested in the following (in addition to other as yet unknown problems):

Aluminum causes constipation and flatulence (your suspicions should be aroused when herbal remedies, dietary changes and/or medications

Minerals

and "natural medications" supplements don't help you). It also causes a tremor in the leg muscle, as well as excessive perspiration, and a loss of strength. The motor nerves can be paralyzed, and there can be a feeling of pins and needles. The absorption of phosphorus (which is necessary for calcium) is reduced, and this leads to bone and brain problems.

Aluminum is found in antacids, which also cause a shortage of vitamins A and B1, and other medications (alumina/magnesia), which also cause a shortage of iron and phosphates. When you take these medications (and you should always avoid doing so), you should also take brewer's yeast, cod-liver oil, (live) yogurt, and acidophilus with digestive enzymes.

Aluminum is also found in aluminum salts of fluorine, which are the enemies of fluorine itself. It is found in processed cheese, in aluminum pots and pans, and in aluminum products such as foil. The use of these objects causes aluminum to penetrate into the body. In summary, the use of cooking utensils and other aluminum products should be avoided entirely, especially in heating or cooking. Use stainless steel, glass, etc. instead. **Consider this a warning!**

Boron

Boron is one of the most recent minerals to date whose importance has been acknowledged.

Boron is found in food (vegetable), as are most of the minerals, and our bodies need small quantities of it. Boron's main property is that it is calcium's glue in the bones. However, in a great deal of research conducted in hospitals and research centers (mainly in the U.S.), the importance of boron in other fields is also being demonstrated.

Research conducted in 1987 indicates the importance of boron during the post-menopausal years, especially in the absorption of other minerals (in men, too). For this reason, it helps in the treatment of osteoporosis, since it enhances and catalyzes metabolic processes.

The need for boron was recognized in 1870, when the subject of borax/boric acid was investigated. For several decades afterwards, this substance was used as a preservative mainly for fish and meat, and, from the beginning of the 20th century, also for vegetables. It was found that in large quantities (as in preservatives), it is harmful, and therefore the use of borates in food for preservative purposes, which was commonplace from the 1920s until the mid-1950s, was prohibited, mainly because of the various additives that converted it into boric acid, until the 1980s. In 1987, its importance was acknowledged once more, **but not as a preservative**.

Minerals

Boron helps with the absorption of calcium, copper, and nitrogen. It increases the libido in post-menopausal women (because of the improvement in the concentration of testosterone in the blood). It helps in the treatment of cancer by enhancing the absorption of the other minerals. Boron helps in the absorption of zinc as well as of vitamin C (ascorbic acid), and has been found to be effective in treating and improving lung function.

Boron negates and prevents negative reactions in estrogen absorption, and in this way helps to reduce calcium loss and the increase in cholesterol and triglycerides as a result of the use of estrogen. It improves the metabolism for the absorption of calcium, and as such constitutes a factor for prevention and/or treatment of osteoporosis and arthritis. Boron raises the testosterone level in the blood threefold, thus enhancing muscle mass. It is necessary for growth (as are other trace minerals such as nickel, silicon, arsenic, cadmium, lithium, vanadium, and so on), apparently not as a direct factor, but rather as a link for calcium and other minerals.

Boron is helpful in curbing memory loss (a side-effect of aging) by stopping electro-encephalographic changes in the brain. It causes an increase in the copper concentration in the brain, as well as in the calcium concentration in the brain and the cortex - thus improving the memory. Boron is active and effective during menopause, especially for hot flashes and night sweats.

There is no daily recommended dietary allowance of boron, but research shows that the body requires no less than 1 mg per day, and up to 30 mg per day as an external supplement. The amount required by our bodies is up to 50 mg, some of which comes from food (if our diet is balanced).

A therapeutic amount of boron is about 3-6 mg, which can be supplied in the form of 25-50 mg of borax decahydrate/sodium tetraborte. This amount is found in a combination supplement/tablet of calcium + magnesium + boron (the boron is 3 mg), and there is also a supplement/tablet of boron (3 mg) alone.

Boron can be found in the following foods: mainly plants, nuts, fruit and legumes, wine, dried fruit (raisins and prunes), broccoli, parsley, almonds, peanuts, apple juice and apple concentrate, cherries, the juice of organic grapes, canned peaches and pears. Boron is found less in animal products such as meat, poultry, fish, and dairy products.

It is easy to supply the body's boron needs (without using external means, except in a therapeutic situation) if the person knows how to plan and consume good (organic) foods.

Toxicity was discovered in research that was conducted on rats, dogs, pigs, and other animals. An amount of about 8 mg per kilogram body weight was found to be toxic (for example, if a person weighs 70 kg and takes 560 mg per day). Bigger amounts were found to cause damage in animals. The maximum amount (according to research) is 500 mg a day, an enormous amount that is almost impossible to consume.

Cadmium

Chemical symbol Cd, specific gravity 8.64, atomic weight 112.4 (cadmium).

Cadmium is a soft, gray-white metal. In nature, it is linked to minerals with zinc. In industry, it is used with other metals; moreover, it regulates the operation of atomic reactors. Cadmium salts are used for manufacturing yellow paints.

Cadmium is a toxic substance that is found in pesticides and enamel coating. It reaches human beings by means of vegetables and grains, mainly, as well as water that has been softened by chemicals, or molluscs and oysters.

Cadmium is considered more toxic than lead, and is found in cigarette smoke, in nickel-cadmium batteries, and in processed coffee products (such as decaffeinated coffee).

The signs of cadmium toxicity include: atherosclerosis, emphysema, and chronic bronchitis; high blood pressure; lung and kidney problems to the point of cancer; heart diseases and problems; and anemia due to a shortage of iron.

You can protect yourself against cadmium toxicity by eating foods that are rich in zinc (such as pumpkin seeds, nuts, and so on), because zinc is a cadmium antagonist; taking vitamin C, which is the specific defense; by avoiding using utensils with enamel coatings (use

Minerals

glass or stainless steel utensils instead); by avoiding white flour products from which the zinc has been extracted (during the whitening process), and only the cadmium remains; if possible, by drinking filtered water or mineral/natural water, and not water from the faucet; by decreasing your consumption of coffee and tea, as cadmium is found in both of them, and by totally avoiding decaffeinated coffee!

Calcium

Chemical symbol Ca, specific gravity 1.55, atomic weight 40.01 (calcium).

Calcium is a metallic chemical element found in our bodies, and one of the most widespread in nature (limestone and chalk are made of calcium). It is gray in color, and creates various compounds easily both in the body and in nature (and in various industries). Calcium is the most important substance for the building of the skeleton and bones: 99% is found in the bones and teeth, and 1% in the soft tissues. It is of enormous importance in the muscles and the heart muscle.

Together with magnesium, calcium regulates the heart rate, and also completes the action of other minerals in the digestive system. Every year, the body "recycles" 20% (one-fifth) of the amount of calcium by releasing calcium from the tissues and the bones and replenishing it from food.

This continuous action does not only occur during menopause, but all our lives, and when our nutrition is poor in (organic) calcium, which must be absorbed back into the bones (which are the reserves of calcium), cumulative damage is caused over the years to the walls of the bones and to the bone itself, which becomes absorbed - and suddenly people become aware of a process that is called "calcium loss."

Minerals

The shortage of calcium can also be caused (and this is the process that occurs generally) when food is rich in phosphorus (too rich, in relation to calcium), and when the diet consists of meat (beef, chicken, and so on), in which the proportion of phosphorus to calcium is opposite to that in human beings - 40 times more!

It is important to know that menopausal vegetarian women lose only 18% of their bone mass, while menopausal carnivorous women lose over 35% - and that is in addition to the loss of calcium over the years prior to menopause.

In order for calcium to be absorbed in the stomach, normal stomach acid (hydrochloride - HCl) is required, as is vitamin D. Its absorption is easier when it comes from unpasteurized dairy products.

The mechanism in a healthy person's stomach contains a "safety" device that prevents the absorption of excessive calcium in the blood, and allows the excess (including the excess from supplements) to pass through harmlessly. When the safety mechanism is defective and there is excessive calcium, problems of calcinosis and hypercalcemia are liable to occur.

In order for calcium to be absorbed in the body and to function properly, calcium - and our bodies - needs magnesium, phosphorus, vitamins A, C, and D, and good proteins.

Absorption occurs mainly in the duodenum (in a short time and at a length of 12 inches only).

Minerals

Calcium problems are likely when the parathyroid hormone is secreted incorrectly, and then an excess of calcium is revealed in blood tests, meaning that calcium is coming out of the bones. This condition must be treated thoroughly.

Calcium influences the action and stimulation of the muscles, and balances potassium and sodium in muscle tension. It is needed for regulating the heart rate, and for the blood coagulation mechanism. Calcium is necessary for transmitting nervous information via nervous impulses, and for activating the hormones that are linked to metabolism. It is important in the metabolism of iron. Calcium safeguards bones and teeth. It is of cardinal importance for the growth of children's bones in general, and for adolescents going through growth spurts. It alleviates growing pains, as well as insomnia.

The recommended dietary allowance of calcium is as follows: for infants of up to 6 months, it is 360 mg, for infants of between 6 and 12 months, it is 540 mg, for children of up to 10 years, it is 800 mg, for youngsters of between 11 and 18 years, it is 1,000 mg, for people over 18 years, it is 800 mg. Pregnant and nursing women should add 400 mg.

People who suffer from backaches, joint problems, difficult menstrual periods, hypoglycemia (lack of sugar), and high blood pressure should take higher doses - under medical supervision, of course.

Calcium is found in the following foods: all

dried herbs, almonds, green leafy vegetables - mainly broccoli and parsley, dried brewer's yeast, filberts, soy flour, dairy products from goats, sheep, and cows, small fish (in the bones), peanuts, soy, dried legumes, sesame paste, and sunflower seeds. Smaller amounts are found in all fruits and vegetables.

If there is a shortage of calcium, the following symptoms are liable to occur: calcium loss - osteoporosis; delayed growth in children; menstrual problems, including lengthy periods/heavy bleeding; nervousness, irritation, poor sleep; poor quality and shape of bones and teeth, leading to leg cramps - tetany; rickets and osteomalacia.

There is toxicity in calcium in daily doses of over 2,000 mg, and with a problematic stomach, there could be a problem of excess - hypercalcemia. This does not include therapeutic cases, in which there is a definite need for more calcium, such as arthritis (and as I mentioned earlier, also in a case where the thyroid gland creates the problem.)

Supplements for calcium are available in the following forms: calcium + magnesium made from dolomite rock; calcium with vitamins to help its absorption; calcium + magnesium, at a proportion of 2:1; calcium + magnesium + boron; and bone meal tablets.

Calcium should be of the lactate type, which originates in milk; or, alternatively, of the gluconate type, which is of plant origin - it is preferable, and is better absorbed in the body.

Chlorine

Chemical symbol Cl, atomic weight 35.46 (chlorum).

Chlorine is a non-metal gas, from the halogen group (chlorine, fluorine, bromide, and iodine). Its color is greenish - hence its name, which comes from the Greek *chloros* - "pale green." It has a pungent odor, and is found in nature in compounds of cooking salt (sodium chloride).

Chlorine is used as a bleach and a disinfectant. It is a mineral that is necessary for nutrition, and serves as an important component in the stomach acid (hydrochloride).

If large quantities are added to the water in swimming pools, children's (and adults') teeth are liable to be destroyed, and the same thing is liable to happen when drinking water has been chlorinated in order to purify it. You should always boil chlorinated water or let it stand for a few hours until the chlorine (which is a gas) evaporates.

Chlorine regulates the acid-base balance in the blood. It works with sodium and potassium as a compound, and helps clean the body by helping the liver's action. It maintains the body's pliancy and muscle tone, and helps convey and distribute the hormones throughout the body. Since it is a component of the stomach acid, it is helpful in digestion, especially of proteins.

The daily recommended dietary allowance for

infants up to 6 months is 0.275-0.7 g, for infants of 6 to 12 months is 0.4-1.2 g, for children of 1-3 years is 0.5-1.5 g, for children of 4-6 years is 0.7-2.1 g, for children of 7-10 years is 0.925-2.775 g, for youngsters of 11-17 years is 1.4-4.2 g, and for people over 18 years is 1.75-5.1 g. It should be noted that in regular nutrition, there is enough salt, which means that there is a regular supply of chlorine, and sometimes even an excess.

Chlorine can be found in the following foods: salt (cooking or sea), seaweed, vegetables (root vegetables contain sodium chloride, leafy vegetables contain potassium chloride), and olives.

People who suffer from high blood pressure (which conventional medicine calls "from an unknown source") are advised to avoid salt and salty foods.

A shortage of chlorine is very rare, unless there is vomiting and/or diarrhea, which expels it, and then it cannot perform its functions. If there is a shortage, it could result in hair and teeth loss.

Chlorine has no toxicity, but daily consumption in excess of 14 g can cause disturbances in the body and lead to unpleasant and toxic side-effects. Even a smaller amount than this can damage the intestinal flora, and impair the production of vitamin B. It may not be toxic, but in large quantities, chlorine disrupts the production of thyroxine, thus weakening the immune system, not to mention that chlorine leads to arteriosclerosis and heart diseases.

Chromium

Chemical symbol Cr, specific gravity 6.7, atomic weight 52.01 (chromium).

Chromium is a hard metal that shines when polished. It is bluish-white in color, and its name derives from the Greek word *chroma*, meaning "color." It is used in the steel industry. Chromium salts are used in the paint, glass, and tanning industries. Chromium is destroyed during the processing of food, and experimental attempts have been made to reintroduce it into food in order to avoid atherosclerosis - a scientific fact that has been proved beyond a shadow of a doubt.

Research has shown that the problem of diabetes is directly linked to nutrition and to a shortage of chromium in the modern diet. Chromium is linked to the regulation of insulin production in the pancreas, and increases its efficiency, so that when there is a shortage of chromium, the pancreas produces low-grade insulin (and a lot of it), thus creating a totally useless strain on the pancreas until its action slows down and finally halts.

The amount of chromium in the body decreases with age, and an interesting phenomenon has been discovered: new-born infants and babies consume a great deal of chromium during pregnancy, which causes their mothers' chromium supply to dwindle.

Minerals

This action does not occur in primitive populations, whose chromium level remains stable in their bodies even during old age - and this is not surprising, since their food is not processed (that is, until "progress" catches up with them).

Chromium always acts in conjunction with other organic factors: with iron, it carries proteins in the blood, and with certain organic links, it is active in the metabolism of sugar; it is called Chromium GTF (glucose tolerant factor) when its activity is not only in the context of diabetes, but also in that of hypoglycemia.

Chromium increases the effectiveness of insulin (both natural and external). It balances the sugars in the body for both diabetes and hypoglycemia. It lowers the levels of cholesterol and fats in the blood, and treats atherosclerosis. It lowers high blood pressure, and helps in growth (in children).

While there are no recommended dietary allowances, the daily amount required for infants of up to 6 months is 0.01-0.04 mg, for children of 6-12 months is 0.02-0.06 mg, for children of 1-3 years is 0.02-0.08 mg, for children of 4-6 years is 0.03-0.12 mg, and for people of 7 and over is 0.05-0.20 mg.

Sometimes, when there is a need for chromium (something that is revealed in hair tests, which show shortages or excesses of minerals and vitamins), it is customary to administer zinc (either alone, or with a chromium

Minerals

supplement), and this improves the chromium situation and the absorption of chromium. A therapeutic dose is much higher than a normal daily amount, and is prescribed by a physician.

Natural chromium tablets, which are suitable for this, are available, as are pure chromium tablets and chromium + selenium tablets. Generally speaking, a sufficient quantity of chromium is found in natural multivitamin and multimineral tablets. People who take brewer's yeast tablets (not torula yeast) obtain chromium from the tablets.

Chromium can be found in the following foods: whole wheat, brown rice, and other whole grains, whole oatmeal porridge, legumes, nuts, dried brewer's yeast, corn oil, meat, and chicken. Fruit and vegetables contain very little chromium.

If there is a shortage of chromium, the following diseases and conditions may occur: diabetes or hypoglycemia, arteriosclerosis, cholesterol/fats and/or heart problems, or even low cholesterol. Remember that a shortage of chromium is linked to a diet of processed food.

Chromium has no known toxicity. Having said that, it must be pointed out that an especially large daily amount of chromium is liable to cause nausea.

Cobalt

Chemical symbol Co, specific gravity 8.90, atomic weight 58.94 (cobaltum).

Cobalt is an extremely heavy metal, similar in color to steel. It is used in the manufacture of especially hard metal tools. Its dark blue color and name are derived from the German word *Kobold* (devil's child), since the German miners thought that it had diabolical and harmful properties.

Cobalt-60 is a radioactive isotope of cobalt, and is used mainly for treating cancerous tissues during radiation therapy. Cobalt is an essential mineral, and it is part of vitamin B_{12}, which is also called cyanocobalamin. It comes mainly from animals, as well as from marine vegetation.

Cobalt is needed for the production of red blood cells, and for the enzymatic system.

Cobalt does not have any toxicity, and there are no daily recommended dietary allowances for it. However, excessive cobalt causes problems in the thyroid gland, something which is extremely rare.

If there is a shortage of cobalt, the phenomena that may occur are identical to those that occur with a shortage of iron or vitamin B_{12}.

Copper

Chemical symbol Cu, specific gravity 8.92, atomic weight 63.57 (cuprum).

Copper is a trace element that is essential for the body, and is found in every cell. It is a soft, reddish-yellow metal that is an excellent conductor of electricity. It is used in the tool industry, especially in the form of bronze or brass.

In the body, it is consumed in milligrams. While the body absolutely cannot be without it, over-consumption is forbidden. Not much is known about copper, but there are many differences of opinion because of the difficulty in investigating it, so I will outline the things that are known for sure.

Copper serves as one of the components that cover, strengthen and insulate the nerve walls with vitamin B (and especially folic acid). It is necessary for the absorption of iron, and essential for its absorption in the blood and its conversion into hemoglobin. Copper is linked to the (positive) oxidation of vitamin C, and to the building of RNA, as well as to the metabolism of proteins. It is necessary for the strengthening of the bones. It is linked to the pigments in the skin and hair (with the amino acid tyrosine.)

There is no daily recommended dietary allowance for copper. The estimated safe daily intake is as follows: for infants up to 6 months, it

Minerals

is 0.5-0.7 mg, for infants of between 6 and 12 months, it is 0.7-1.0 mg, for children of between 1 and 3 years, it is 1.0-1.5 mg, for children of between 4 and 6 years, it is 1.5-2.0 mg, for children of between 7 and 10 years, it is 2.0-2.5 mg, and for people of 11 years and over, it is 2.0-3.0 mg.

The amount of copper should be increased if there is a consumption of zinc: for every extra 50 mg of zinc, 2 mg of copper should be added, since these two minerals "compete" with each other, but both are necessary.

Copper is found in the following foods: whole grains (whole wheat, brown rice, and so on), buckwheat, dried brewer's yeast, molasses, mushrooms, walnuts, lentils, and green leafy vegetables.

Copper is not destroyed easily, and correct nutrition is sufficient to ensure the right amount of it.

If there is a shortage of copper, the following symptoms may occur: calcium loss, anemia, and general weakness; respiratory problems and edemas; nervous disorders (because of the damage to the myelin - the nerve covering); sores on the skin, and hair loss.

Copper toxicity is extremely rare, unless it is taken in enormous quantities. Unnecessary copper supplements occur in places where there are copper water pipes, and copper cooking utensils are used.

In most cases, copper is found in multimineral

and multivitamin formulas or tablets, and there is hardly any need to take it separately (except in a therapeutic situation, under medical supervision).

Excess copper has been found in people who suffer from mental depression.

Fluorine

Chemical symbol F, specific gravity 1.69, atomic weight 9 (fluorine).

Fluorine is a mineral that is found in every tissue in the body. It is essential especially for bones and teeth, in that it helps calcium to be absorbed in the necessary places. Excessive fluorine is toxic (to the point of death), and when it is found in water at a proportion of more than 2 parts per million, it harms the teeth, causing them to appear spotty.

Fluorine is found in two forms:

Calcium fluoride - its natural form (and the one that is necessary for the body).

Sodium fluoride - its synthetic (and toxic) form, whose addition to drinking water is highly controversial.

The gigantic metal companies are guilty of lobbying for the use of synthetic fluoride (which is a by-product of the steel industry), because in this way, they spare themselves the bother of having to find a place to store it.

Fluoride must not be taken as a supplement, unless prescribed by a physician, and even then, it must be used in its natural form.

An amount of over 20 mg a day is toxic.

If there is a shortage of fluorine, there can be problems and weakness in the bones and teeth. If there is an excess (toxicity) of fluorine, the following symptoms may occur: problems and weakness in the teeth (spotty teeth); the destruction of phosphatase, which is the enzyme that is important in the metabolism of vitamins; damage to the brain tissue - in places where the water is rich in fluoride, there is an increase in the percentage of children with Down's syndrome; damage to the bones - research has shown that people who live in areas where the water is rich in fluorides (fluorinated water, to which fluorine has been added), there is a higher percentage of bone fractures in the elderly.

In this case, calcium protects against the toxicity of fluorine.

Minerals

Iodine

Chemical symbol I, atomic weight 126.9 (iodum).

Iodine is a non-metal, chemical element from the halogen group (chlorine, fluorine, bromide, and iodine). Its color is deep purple, and hence its name, which comes from the word *ioeides* - "violet-colored" in Greek. Every body needs iodine. Iodine salts are used in the photographic industry and in medicine.

The general amount that is found in our body is about 10-25 mg, and most of it is in the thyroid gland. This means that a minor shortage of iodine can cause problems in the thyroid gland (which is found in the front part of the throat), leading to problems with metabolism in the cells of the tissues, with the regulation of digestion, and with the regulation of heat in the body. A slowing-down of metabolism (in the activity of the thyroid gland) results in a slowing-down of or decrease in hormone production, sensitivity to cold, fatigue and drowsiness, apathy, and weight-gain, since iodine constitutes an integral part of the hormone thyroxine, which is the principal hormone of the thyroid gland, and it has additional actions: converting carotene into vitamin A, absorption of carbohydrates in the small intestine, and the digestion and burning of fats.

In the form of a medication, iodine can be

Minerals

dangerous, but there is no risk when it appears in food. There are foods that contain anti-thyroxine substances, and decrease the action of iodine, such as the cabbage family (if eaten in large quantities) and mustard seeds.

Iodine prevents the rise of blood-fats, and arteriosclerosis. Furthermore, it promotes correct growth, improves learning, and enhances and accelerates thought processes (mental agility). It improves general energy, and controls and balances weight (by burning excess fat) - and for this reason is good for dieting. Iodine is helpful for the growth and maintenance of healthy hair, nails, teeth, and skin.

The daily recommended dietary allowance for infants up to the age of 6 months is 40 mcg, for infants up to the age of 1 year is 50 mcg, for children of between 1 and 3 years is 70 mcg, for children of between 4 and 6 years is 90 mcg, for children of between 7 and 10 years is 120 mcg, and for people of 11 onward is 150 mcg. Pregnant women should take 25 mcg more, and nursing women should take 50 mcg more. Therapeutic doses are higher - sometimes six or ten times higher - but only under medical supervision.

Iodine is found in the following foods: seaweed (fresh or in tablet form), marine fish, sea food, vegetables, and onions grown in iodine-rich soil

The major part of iodine supplement during the therapeutic period (such as during a diet for losing weight) will be in the form of seaweed tablets, or from cooking seaweed and drinking it.

If there is a shortage of iodine, the following symptoms may occur: goiter, a disease of the thyroid gland; weight-gain, or alternatively difficulty in losing weight; psychological and mental disturbances; impaired release of energy, leading to sluggishness; a lower body temperature, which can indicate hypo-activity (under-activity) of the thyroid gland; and lastly, coarse, dry skin.

Comment: Sometimes, when there is a shortage of iodine (not even a serious shortage), there is a slowing-down of the action of the thyroid gland. Even if blood tests apparently show that the hormone level is normal (within the parameters), we know from experience that in almost everyone whose weight is higher than normal, his/her thyroid gland is working **too slowly** (too slowly in relation to his/her weight).

The only time there is toxicity in iodine is when synthetic iodine supplements are taken (as medications). There is no toxicity in natural supplements to food, but in very large quantities, hyperactivity and nervousness can occur. Sometimes there are people who are allergic to iodine, and most of them have a history of a use of medical iodine for tests and X-rays.

Iron

Chemical symbol Fe, specific gravity 7.87, atomic weight 55.8 (ferrum).

Iron is a chemical element. It is the metal that has been most commonly used for thousands of years, and is (almost) not found in nature in its pure form.

Iron is a mineral that is necessary for life, and it belongs to the group of minerals that must be consumed in small quantities. (Just to remind you - the second group must be consumed in large quantities, including magnesium and calcium.)

More than half of the iron in the body is used as a compound in the red blood cells (hemoglobin) together with protein and copper, and it also participates in the creation of myoglobin, which is the protein that stores oxygen in the muscle (in the red color).

Iron is found in every cell in the body. For its assimilation in the body (and its transport) vitamin C, folic acid, vitamin E, copper, manganese, and cobalt are required, and there must be a balance with calcium and phosphorus and with the rest of the vitamin B complex. For its absorption, the presence of hydrochloric acid (HCl) in the stomach is necessary, and a digestive protein that regulates its absorption via the mucous membranes.

Iron and calcium constitute the primary

nutrient deficiencies in women, and in order not to reach the point of deficiency, nutrients for several basic processes must be provided. Remember that during a single month, women lose **double** the amount of iron that men do.

Iron renews itself in the body naturally, and red blood cells renew themselves every four months (120 days). For this to occur, there must be balance, as I mentioned above.

There are several points to remember about iron:

Its absorption in the body is less than 5%; therefore, during the course of a day, an amount no smaller than 400 mg of iron (organic) must be consumed in order for the required amount to be absorbed.

Drinking regular tea reduces the absorption of iron by between a third and a half because of the tannic acid in it, and drinking coffee after a meal reduces the absorption of iron by more than a third.

Preservatives and anti-oxidants in food, such as BHTA, phosphatase, or EDTA, prevent the absorption of iron (as well as the rest of the minerals, especially zinc and magnesium).

When there is a need for iron supplements (in tablet form) for people who suffer from anemia or low hemoglobin, or for pregnant women, they must demand organic iron whose absorption and assimilation are better than the ferrous sulfate (which is not organic) that is supplied by the drug companies (mainly), and sometimes **also** cause constipation and nausea, and damage the vitamin E in the body.

In pernicious anemia, iron with the addition of B complex and especially B12 is needed. In leukemia or colitis, iron is needed, and it must be remembered that with problems such as cirrhosis of the liver and diabetes (that derives from impaired functioning of the pancreas), iron deposits can form as a result of taking excessive doses. In cases of sickle-cell anemia or hemochromatosis or thalassemia, iron must not be taken in a concentrated form, and sometimes another mineral (such as zinc) is required in order to treat the problem.

The roles of iron include: curing and preventing anemia, increasing energy by reducing fatigue, improving the color of the blood (and the color of children's cheeks), helping growth in children, improving resistance to disease, and improving the transport of oxygen in the blood to the cells.

The recommended dietary allowance of iron for infants up to 6 months is 10 mg, for children of between 6 months and 3 years is 15 mg, for children of between 4 and 10 years is 10 mg, for males of between 11 and 18 years is 18 mg, and for adult males is 10 mg. For females of between 11 and 50, the amount is 18 mg; above 50, it is 10 mg. Pregnant and lactating women should add between 30 and 60 mg.

Iron can be found in the following foods: dried vegetables and herbs, dried brewer's yeast, whole sesame seed and whole sesame paste, molasses, soy flour, dried legumes (chickpeas, fava beans, lentils, black-eyed peas), fish, cashew nuts, pine nuts, almonds, peanuts, calf liver (be careful of hormones and antibiotics), meat (the inner organs), green leafy vegetables, and chicken.

Meat: You should eat "organic" meat, that is, meat that does not contain hormones and antibiotics, substances that cause damage to the human body, such as hormonal upsets, especially in women.

The amount of iron in (natural) multivitamin tablets is sufficient for the daily requirement, but not for therapeutic purposes.

If there is a shortage of iron, the following symptoms may occur: anemia, a shortage of red blood cells, a low rate of red-blood-cell formation, a decline in the blood supply to the cells, especially to the muscles, depression and lack of appetite, a slowing down of cerebral activity (impaired memory), weakness, vertigo, pallor, hair loss, and shortness of breath.

Toxicity is rare, unless iron is taken during illnesses (as I listed before), or a daily dosage of over 100 mg is taken over an extended period.

It must be remembered that non-organic iron is supplied in amounts larger than 100 mg in the knowledge that only 10% of it will be absorbed in the body, and for this reason, it is preferable to consume only natural iron.

Minerals

Lead

Chemical symbol Pb, specific gravity 11.34, atomic weight 20.721 (plumbum).

Lead is a soft, rust-resistant metal that is used for pipes, soldering, and casting (of characters in printing).

If lead reaches the bone, it replaces the calcium; for this reason, calcium-rich food will help in avoiding the absorption of lead.

Lead poisoning is becoming an ecological disease that is developing very rapidly. In addition to exhaust fumes that are rich in lead, people absorb lead from smoking and passive smoking. Lead poisoning can be fatal to human beings, even in small quantities, which is why gasoline is now sold in an unleaded form. Moreover, lead is being removed from commercial paints and children's paints, from ceramics, and so on. Lead and its toxicity accumulate in the body, and, as can be seen from the list of symptoms, it is difficult to identify lead poisoning as the cause.

The signs of lead poisoning include: multiple sclerosis - neuro-muscular diseases; stomachaches, vertigo, and headaches; hyperactivity in children; anemia, nervousness, fatigue, and loss of appetite; damage to the liver, kidneys, and heart; partial paralysis of the limbs; blindness and mental disturbances (from the accumulation of lead in the head); problems in the reproductive system (and impotence in men); and impaired growth in infants and children whose mothers suffered from lead poisoning;.

You can protect yourself from lead poisoning by consuming the following: calcium, vitamin D (in combination with calcium); vitamin C in therapeutic daily doses of at least 1,000-3,000 mg; vitamin B1, which is especially valuable for this; at least 25,000 International Units of vitamin A; lecithin, potassium iodide that binds to the lead in the body and helps to excrete it; legumes, beans, and algin from seaweed (in powder form).

Minerals

Magnesium

Chemical symbol Mg, specific gravity 1.74, atomic weight 24.3 (magnesium).

Magnesium is a light metallic, chemical element that burns with a very strong light. Its color is white (silver). In industry, it is combined with aluminum, and it is used in the aircraft industry and in medicine.

Magnesium is one of the most important minerals in the human body, and it operates with and complements calcium in the building of bones and muscles. Magnesium is found in nerve fluids, and causes muscle fibers to release tension, while calcium stimulates the muscle fibers to contract. This action also occurs in the heart, which is a muscle. The calcium contracts the muscle, and the magnesium contributes to its release and regulates the heartbeat.

Both magnesium and calcium constitute a component in the gums. Only in recent years has magnesium been "acknowledged" by the medical establishment (while in homeopathic medicine, it has been known as a positive factor for years). The total amount of magnesium in the body is slightly more than 20 grams, and it is a mineral that helps the body under conditions of stress. Research has revealed that children who suffer from convulsions and nervous disorders must take more magnesium, and milk must be omitted from their diets, because the fluorides in

Minerals

milk bind to the magnesium and remove it. People who eat refined or processed foods (such as refined carbohydrates or alcohol) must increase their magnesium intake, as must people who take diuretics, or women who take oral contraceptives. Low quantities of magnesium in the body lead to destructive diseases (including cancer).

Magnesium is an antacid and counteracts the stomach acid, so it should not be taken with or soon after a meal containing protein (that requires stomach acid), or early in the morning.

Magnesium is necessary for the absorption of calcium and the assimilation of vitamin C, as well as for the conversion of blood sugar into energy. It activates enzymatic systems that require various biological actions, and is essential for maintaining RNA/DNA. It is necessary for the synthesis of several amino acids, as well as for dissolving kidney stones (with vitamin B6), and for the normal contraction of the muscles. Magnesium also gets rid of body odor and halitosis (as do zinc, vitamin B6 and PABA). It is important for maintaining the health of the gums, and is necessary for the regulation of body fluids (swelling in the face, joints, etc.), and for regulating the heartbeat rate. Magnesium alleviates heartburn (as an antacid), digestive problems and pains, and helps to combat depression.

The daily recommended dietary allowance of magnesium for infants up to 6 months old is 50

Minerals

mg, for infants of between 6 and 12 months is 70 mg, for children of between 1 and 3 years is 150 mg, for children of between 4 and 6 years is 200 mg, for children of between 7 and 10 years is 250 mg. For males of between 11 and 14 years, the RDA is 350 mg, for males of between 15 and 18 years it is 400 mg, and over that age is 350 mg. For females of over 11 years, the RDA is 300 mg, while pregnant and nursing women should take an additional 150 mg (under medical supervision, of course).

Children whose diet contains a lot of protein must increase their intake, and those who consume milk must increase their intake of magnesium-rich food. Adults who consume alcohol, milk and dairy products, and proteins must increase their magnesium intake.

Magnesium is found in the following foods: most fruits and vegetables such as figs, citrus fruit, apples (especially dark green ones), in dried herbs, soy flour, nuts, almonds, molasses, brewer's yeast, buckwheat, legumes (especially black-eyed peas), whole wheat, brown rice, oatmeal, cornstarch, dried onions, and millet.

Magnesium is present in natural tablets that are combined with vitamin B6, as well as in natural tablets/chealates or combined with calcium (at a proportion of 1:2) or combined with calcium + boron.

If there is a shortage of magnesium, the following symptoms may occur: atherosclerosis, high blood pressure, irregular heartbeat, calcium stones - especially in people whose consumption of dairy products is high, over-stimulation of muscles and nerves, nervous tics and contractions, convulsions, and fits.

There is toxicity only when taken in very large doses over a long time. A daily dosage of 30 grams or more has been found to be harmful.

The body absorbs only about a third of the amount of magnesium that it consumes, so that no less than 120 mg must be taken in order to ensure the minimal amount (this is much less than a harmful amount).

Minerals

Manganese

Chemical symbol Mn, specific gravity 7.3, atomic weight 54.93 (manganium).

Manganese is a hard, brittle element. It has a silvery color, and is used in combination with iron in order to obtain superior steel. In the lighting industry, it is used for yellow lighting. In the body, its action is complex, which makes research about it difficult. In recent years, additional information pertaining to manganese has emerged, but since there are still no medications for problems caused by a shortage of manganese, no conclusions have been reached yet.

The body secretes 4-5 mg of manganese every day, which is the minimal daily amount. It has been found that a larger quantity of manganese is required for meat-eaters and consumers of dairy products, since the exaggerated amounts of calcium and phosphorus impair the absorption of manganese.

Manganese helps the pancreas in its function and in the correct use of glucose. It serves as a component of the bones (as a collagen supplement), as well as the glue that binds calcium, magnesium, and phosphorus. It is active in the production of thyroxine (the thyroid gland's hormone), and sex hormones. It is important in the production of cholesterol and in the breakdown and composition of fats. It

Minerals

strengthens the bone cartilage, as well as the points where the muscles are joined to the bones. It serves as a component in the nervous system (a neurotransmitter, acetylcholine). It plays a role in the enzymes for the absorption of vitamin B1, biotin, vitamin C, and choline, as well as in the prevention of sterility. With lecithin, it improves the memory and concentration, and reduces stress.

No daily recommended dietary allowance has been established. The estimated safe daily intake is as follows: For infants of up to 6 months, it is 0.5-0.7 mg, for infants of between 7 and 12 months, it is 0.7-1.0 mg, for children of between 1 and 3 years, it is 1.0-1.5 mg, for children of between 4 and 6 years, it is 1.5-2.0 mg, for children of between 7 and 10 years, it is 2.0-3.0 mg, and for people over 11 years, it is 2.5-5.0 mg.

If large amounts of dairy products and meat are consumed, larger quantities of manganese are required.

Manganese is contained in natural multimineral and multivitamin tablets and formulas.

Manganese is found in the following foods: mainly in whole grains (brown rice, whole wheat, etc,), egg yolks, walnuts, almonds, peanuts, green leafy vegetables, peas, beets, avocado, barley, whole oats, and in most vegetables and fruits (that have not undergone industrial processes).

If there is a shortage of manganese, the

following symptoms may occur: multiple sclerosis, soft bones, weakness in ligaments and tendons; weakness in the muscles (a lack of muscular coordination - ataxia or myasthenia gravis - serious muscle weakness); disrupted nerve actions and mental confusion; sexual indifference; recurring vertigo; digestive disorders, and impaired metabolism (connected to the thyroid gland); an increase in blood sugar; slow growth and development.

Manganese toxicity is extremely rare, and is liable to be created by industrial toxins. As a rule, there is no need to take too much of it.

Minerals

Mercury

Chemical symbol Hg, specific gravity 14.2, atomic weight 200.6 (hydrargyrum).

Mercury is a heavy metallic chemical element that is found in nature in a liquid form (at a normal temperature). The color of mercury resembles that of silver, and it is used in thermometers and other scientific instruments. As a chemical compound in nitric acid and alcohol, it is used for filling detonators, fuses, and mercury-detonated bullets.

Mercury is poisonous to human beings, and as a result of the dumping of industrial waste, it is found in lakes and rivers in the form of a substance called methyl-mercury, and that is how it gets into fishes and from there into people.

Fungicidal sprays for foodstuffs contain mercury, and this is another way in which mercury gets into the human body. There are also medications that contain mercury chloride, which contributes to the accumulation of mercury in the body.

Signs of hydrargyrism (mercury poisoning) include: damage to the brain and the central nervous system; disturbances of enzymatic actions in the body; damage to the kidneys and liver, to the point of blindness and paralyses; tremors, mental degeneration, diarrhea, and speech difficulties.

In order to defend ourselves against mercury,

Minerals

the following are recommended: dried brewer's yeast, since it contains selenium (see "Selenium"); calcium, since it neutralizes almost all poisons (see "Calcium"); lecithin and hydrochloride; taking vitamins from the antioxidant group on a daily basis (A, B, C, E); refraining from eating food that has been sprayed with insecticides, and from drinking unfiltered water from the faucet.

Molybdenum

Chemical symbol Mo, specific gravity 0.2, atomic weight 42 (molybdenum).

There is very little information about the trace mineral molybdenum. It is a component of several enzymes, and it is linked to the production of red blood cells, as well as to the metabolism of fats and carbohydrates.

Molybdenum helps to extract the iron from its storage places in the liver, and is active in fighting anemia. It promotes a general feeling of good health. It has an effect that prevents tooth decay.

There is no daily recommended dietary allowance for molybdenum, but the estimated safe daily intake is as follows: For infants of up to 6 months, it is 0.03-0.06 mg, for infants of between 6 and 12 months, it is 0.04-0.06 mg, for children of between 1 and 3 years, it is 0.05-0.10 mg, for children of between 4 and 6 years, it is 0.06-0.15 mg, for children of between 7 and 10 years, it is 0.10-0.30 mg, and for people of 11 years and over, it is 0.15-0.50 mg.

Molybdenum is contained in most natural multivitamin and multimineral formulas.

Molybdenum is found in the following foods: whole grains, dark vegetables, and legumes. The molybdenum content depends on the quality of the soil.

The symptoms of a shortage of molybdenum are unknown.

Minerals

Molybdenum's toxicity is unknown, but huge quantities are liable to cause a shortage of copper, something that is extremely rare. Special attention should be paid to molybdenum only in cases of the entire diet consisting of processed food, and completely lacking in nutritional value.

Nickel

Chemical symbol Ni, specific gravity 8.90, atomic weight 58.69 (nickel).

Nickel is a hard, white, shiny metal that does not rust, and it is therefore used in the production process of metals and steel. Its name is derived from the German word *Kupfer-nickel*.

Nickel's main functions have not yet been finally clarified, even though we know that it activates a number of enzymatic systems in the body, and is found in high concentrations in RNA.

This is one of the groups of trace metals that is necessary for us in small amounts, and since it is found in mainly in vegetables, it is not problematic. Apparently, it is not necessary as a separate supplement.

Nickel toxicity occurs only through industrial poisons.

There are no nickel supplements, and it is not contained in vitamin or mineral tablets, since its main functions have not yet been defined, and the required amount seems to be found in food.

Phosphorus

Chemical symbol P, atomic weight 13 (phosphorus).

Phosphorus is common in a compound form in nature, since it is found in every living cell.

The mineral is found in two forms: the white form that is highly flammable, hence the name *phos*, which means "light," and *phor*, which means "carrier" (in Greek); and the red form, which is stable.

The phosphorus compounds are phosphates - chemical fertilizers.

Phosphorus operates together with calcium. In the bones, there is more calcium and less phosphorus, and in the soft tissues, the opposite is true. Phosphorus is involved with and linked to the chemical actions of all the cells.

Phosphorus is important for the absorption of vitamins B2 and B3, and it plays a part in the metabolism of carbohydrates and fats. Moreover, it is significant for growth and heredity. It is an important component of phospholipids (such as lecithin), which are crucial for the breakdown of fats and the cholesterol balance, and it is also important for normal hormonal secretion.

Pregnant women are advised to take more phosphorus than normal, and in the proportion of phosphorus to calcium (1 phosphorus to 25 calcium), it must be remembered that children need more calcium, and care must be taken not to upset the balance.

There is a direct link between the consumption of phosphorus (from food) and the state of the bones and calcium loss, and that is because meat contains 40 times more phosphorus than calcium!

University studies that have investigated osteoporosis have found that in women who are vegetarians (and consume eggs and dairy products), calcium loss is only about half of what it is in carnivorous women, who lose calcium from the bones to the tune of 35%, and this loss weakens the bones. The processed food industry uses phosphorus (mainly in the form of a compound with sodium), which causes the amount of phosphorus that is consumed by the body to be higher than what it should be.

For instance, baking powder contains phosphorus and sodium salt, which gives flour a whiter color. (Phosphorus and calcium salt is more balanced.) Preservatives are connected to phosphoric acid in that those kinds of compounds make it difficult for bacteria to reproduce. Phosphorus salt is added to raw meat that is not fresh (or to salty cheeses) in order to disguise the unpleasant odor.

Another example is soft drinks, which, in addition to food colorings, also include phosphorus, giving them a slightly sour taste, and also increasing the life-span of the bubbles of gas. However, it washes away the calcium in the digestive system, and prevents the absorption of magnesium in the blood by means of a compound that is not absorbable. The study that revealed these facts also showed that damage is caused to the zinc balance.

The salt imbalance that is caused by eating processed foods (white and nice-looking) and drinking soft drinks destroys every healthy part,, and for this reason, you should read labels to see if phosphorus appears as sodium phosphate, calcium phosphate or sodium pyrophosphate.

Phosphorus accelerates the healing of bone fractures, and other fractures and damage. It promotes growth, and contributes to the strengthening of teeth and gums. It reduces the pains of arthritis, and increases the energy for studying and athletic activity by means of the metabolism of fats and carbohydrates. Phosphorus is a component of myelin - the substance that constitutes the nerve sheaths that transmit nervous impulses. It halts the level of acidity in the body.

It should be noted that aluminum and excessive iron and magnesium render phosphorus ineffective.

The daily recommended amount for infants up to 2 months is 240-500 mg, for infants up to 1 year is 360-500 mg, for children up to 3 years is 500-800 mg, for children up to 10 years is 800-1,000 mg, and for youngsters up to 18 years is 1,000-1,200 mg. The daily recommended dietary allowance for adults is 800-1,200 mg, with the higher amount recommended for pregnant or nursing women.

Minerals

Phosphorus can be found in the following foods: fish, chicken, beef, eggs, whole grains, nuts, sunflower seeds, pumpkin seeds, and sesame seeds. Remember that the foods that are richer in phosphorus than they are in calcium (besides the various kinds of meat) are: avocado, nuts and almonds, eggs, sunflower seeds, bananas, lecithin, wheat-germ and bran, soy, brewer's yeast, legumes, lentils, and mushrooms.

It is highly recommended - especially after age 40 - to cut down on the consumption of all kinds of meat, and to increase the amount of green leafy vegetables, since after this age, there are problems with the absorption of excess phosphorus by the kidneys.

If there is a shortage of phosphorus, the following symptoms may occur: weak bones and teeth (weakness in the gums), rickets, arthritis, respiratory problems, fatigue (including mental fatigue), and pus in the body and in the gums.

Phosphorus is not known to be toxic, but excessive amounts of it harm other balances, as was explained above (especially calcium).

Minerals

Potassium

Chemical symbol K (not to be confused with vitamin K), specific gravity 0.86, atomic weight 39.096 (kalium).

Potassium is a metal that is not found freely in nature, but rather in various compounds. Potassium works in conjunction with sodium for the balance and regulation of the body's fluids, since potassium is found in most of the fluids in the cells (the intracellular fluid), and the major amount of sodium is found in the intercellular or extracellular fluid. They operate together to regulate the heartbeat. As long as the person does not take diuretics or cortisones, and does not suffer from kidney diseases or diarrhea and vomiting, potassium will be supplied naturally by his diet.

Many of the actions of potassium are performed in conjunction with another mineral, as we stated above. Potassium also works with calcium to regulate the nervous activity of the muscles, and with phosphorus to regulate the brain. Excessive salt in food stemming from the consumption of salty foods or the addition of a lot of salt to food, causes a loss of potassium, resulting in edemas (swellings), irregular heartbeat, and muscle damage. Sometimes, it is also an important factor in high blood pressure; tea, coffee, and alcohol, as well as drastic weight reduction have the same effect.

Minerals

The functions of potassium include stimulating nervous impulses that activate the muscles to contract and to flex. Moreover, potassium is necessary for growth and for cell metabolism. It regulates the body fluids (together with sodium), and is required for maintaining their alkalinity. Potassium activates and stimulates the kidneys, and maintains the adrenal glands, which are responsible for fatigue and allergies. Potassium plays an important part in the process of transforming glucose into glycogen. It is connected with conveying oxygen to the brain, and is important for the balance (and lowering) of blood pressure. Finally, potassium is important for the health of the skin.

While there is no daily recommended dietary allowance of potassium, infants up to one year should have 350-1,300 mg, while children over one year should have up to 2,000 mg.

In conditions of stress or sugar problems, or when consuming sugars, the amounts should be increased.

Adults should have 2,000-2,500 mg per day. People who drink coffee, tea, or alcohol should increase the amount, as should those with sugar and blood pressure problems, or those who take diuretics or who are on a carbohydrate-free diet.

Potassium can be found in the following foods: all dried herbs, sunflower seeds, dried onion and garlic, dried fruits, dried legumes, nuts, yams, mushrooms, all vegetables (especially green leafy vegetables), bananas, and all the other vegetables and fruit, cereal plants and fish. It is recommended that people who lack potassium in their bodies, and suffer from tension and cramps in their muscles before jogging or exercise drink a glass of citrus juice in order to get some potassium.

If there is a lack of potassium, the person could suffer from hypoglycemia (a shortage of sugar) that is followed by diarrhea; edemas (accumulation of fluids); constipation and irregularity, or diarrhea; impaired muscle and nerve functioning; various allergies; or tachycardia (abnormally rapid heartbeat).

Similar symptoms can be caused when there is a shortage of magnesium or vitamin B.

Over 25,000 mg of potassium chloride can cause toxicity (this amount is way above the recommended daily amount), so potassium hardly ever causes toxicity.

Selenium

Chemical symbol Se, specific gravity 4.82, atomic weight 78.96 (selenium).

Discovered about 30 years ago, selenium is one of the newer members of the trace element group. It is a non-metallic, chemical element that converts radiation energy (light) into electrical energy easily. This is the origin of its name - *selene* ("moon" in Greek). For this reason, it is used in the preparation of photo-electric cells. Its action in the body is different.

Selenium retards aging; it is an excellent antioxidant and expels radicals from the body. Thus, it **fortifies the immune system** and reduces heart attacks.

Research has shown that there is an inverse relation between contracting cancer and selenium, and that cancer patients have been found to have a very low level of selenium in their blood. Moreover, in regions that are poor in selenium (in food), three times more cases of liver diseases, reproductive disorders, and heart diseases (in children, too) have been found than in selenium-rich areas.

Today, because of chemical fertilizers (sprays), the amount of selenium in the earth has decreased or even disappeared altogether. This phenomenon requires the consumption of selenium supplements. Its vegetable sources (which are its main ones) are onions, garlic, and

Minerals

the seeds of whole wheat that was grown in earth that was not fertilized with chemicals and not sprayed - that is, organic.

Selenium is destroyed in industrial food processing.

Selenium prevents and cures various kinds of cancer. It is an anti-oxidant 100 times more powerful than vitamin E. It is synergistic with vitamin E (that is, it completes and strengthens it) and distributes the vitamin in the body, thus creating antibodies for the immune system. It breaks down and purifies toxic chemical compounds and heavy metals. It prevents lead, cadmium, and mercury poisoning, and gets rid of mercury toxicity. It helps to create hard protein compounds, thus helping hair and nails. It is helpful in maintaining the beauty and elasticity of the skin and the hair, and prevents dandruff. It maintains the normal state of the muscles (including the heart muscle). It is important for the treatment of allergies caused by environmental pollution (in therapeutic doses). It decreases hot flashes and other problems of menopause. It helps to prevent heart diseases.

There is no daily recommended dietary allowance for selenium. The estimated safe daily intake is as follows: for infants of up to 6 months, it is 0.01-0.04 mg, for infants of between 6 and 12 months, it is 0.02-0.06 mg, for children of between 1 and 3 years, it is 0.02-0.08 mg, for children of between 4 and 6 years, it is

Minerals

0.03-0.12 mg, for children of between 7 and 10 years, it is 0.05-0.20 mg, for people of 11 years and over, it is 0.06-0.20 mg. Children should not be administered therapeutic doses, as selenium is liable to take the place of fluorine.

Selenium is found in the following foods: onions, bean sprouts, tomatoes, broccoli, whole grains and wheat germ (that were not sprayed with chemicals), marine fish and sea food, and brewer's yeast (not torula yeast).

If there is a shortage of selenium, the following symptoms may occur: low resistance to disease; a greater susceptibility to malignant diseases; muscle diseases and muscle weakness throughout the body (including the heart muscle); degenerative liver diseases; general reproductive disorders; atherosclerosis, high blood pressure.

Generally speaking, there is no fear of toxicity because of the lack of selenium in food; having said that, toxicity can result from very high doses that are not part of a supervised treatment. In therapeutic doses, when there is a shortage of selenium in the body (as in the case of cancer), higher therapeutic doses are generally given.

Silicon

Chemical symbol Si, specific gravity 2.33, atomic weight 28.06 (silicium).

Silicon is a non-metallic, chemical element. It is gray in color, and crystalline in structure. It is the main element in the world of rocks and minerals of which the crust of the earth is composed. It occurs naturally as silicate (a salt of silicic acid).

Until recent years, it was thought that since it is the most common element, there is no danger of a shortage, but tests reveal that silicon shortages occur in the body, mainly because of poor nutrition, lacking in minerals (junk food), which leads to symptoms of shortage.

If there is a shortage of silicon, the following symptoms may occur: skin problems; bone weakness; hair problems (mainly hair loss); nail problems (mainly split nails).

No toxicity of silicon has been found, and there are no daily recommended dietary allowances. Silicon is found in plants (such as horse-tail). If there are signs of a lack of silicon, or if tests (such as hair tests) reveal a shortage, silicon must be taken as a supplement for a long time. Experience has shown that a reasonable period of time for seeing positive results (after the absorption of silicon in the body) is between three months and a year.

Sodium

Chemical symbol Na, specific gravity 0.97, atomic weight 23 (natrium).

Sodium is a soft metal, with a silvery color and shine that quickly disappears upon exposure to air because of its tendency to oxidize rapidly.

Sodium is found in the extracellular fluid in our bodies: blood and lymph. In contrast, potassium is found in the intracellular fluid, and the two elements have to work together in a balanced way. Both of them maintain the fluid balance of the body, while sodium together with chlorine maintain the acid-base balance. This is done by means of a regulating mechanism in the body, which works as follows: chlorine is secreted when there is a tendency toward acidity, and sodium is secreted when there is a tendency toward alkalinity.

Since the daily sodium consumption in our modern world is far more than the body's minimum requirements, there is more to say about problems and diseases caused by an excess of sodium than by a lack of it.

Sodium is necessary for normal nerve action, and for maintaining the tension of the taunus muscles, together with potassium. It maintains the acid-base balance in the body, that is, the regulation of acidity. It maintains the body fluids and is necessary for the production of hydrochloride in the stomach. It looks after the

Minerals

blood, and is responsible for keeping the calcium and other minerals in it.

There is no daily recommended dietary allowance for sodium. The estimated safe daily intake is as follows: For infants up to the age of 6 months, it is 0.115-0.35 g, for infants of between 6 and 12 months, it is 0.25-0.75 g, for children of between 1 and 3 years, it is 0.325-0.975 g, for children of between 4 and 6 years, it is 0.45-1.35 g, for children of between 7 and 10 years, it is 0.60-1.80 g, for youngsters of between 11 and 17 years, it is 0.90-2.270 mg, and for people of 18 and over, it is 1.10-3.30 mg.

Something you should know: Sometimes a craving for salt is a result of insufficient adrenal gland function because of a shortage of the hormone that oversees the accumulation of sodium (it controls the salt).

Sodium can be found in the following foods: all vegetables, proteins, eggs, dried brewer's yeast, sesame seeds, legumes, goat's and sheep's milk, whole grains, nuts, white cheeses, dried fruits, and nearly all fruit. It is found in smaller quantities in dairy products such as yogurt, etc. Table salt or cooking salt are pure sodium chloride, and they supply too much sodium. It is preferable to use pure sea salt, as well as root vegetables such as beets and celery (which is used as a "medication" for high blood pressure).

If there is a shortage of sodium, the following symptoms may occur: Impaired digestion of

Minerals

carbohydrates; flatulence; dehydration; an accumulation of acidity in the body, resulting in arthritis, rheumatism, etc.; neuralgia; loss of muscle weight; impaired function of the adrenal glands, leading to problems and difficulties in withstanding pressures.

The symptoms of a shortage of sodium are liable to manifest themselves in people who refrain from using all kind of salt (including sea salt).

Since sodium is a component of salt (NaCl), most people have an **excess** of sodium, and that is because the use of salt is widespread.

All processed and ready-made foods contain salt or monosodium glutamate (I highly recommend that you stay away from that substance), and sodium is also found in baking powder, baking soda, and so on.

Excessive sodium turns into caustic soda, which is liable to cause cancer following the stimulation of the tissues.

Because of the body's (and especially the kidneys') attempt to get rid of the excess sodium via the urine, impaired kidney function occurs, as do high blood pressure, edemas, and blurred vision.

Strontium

Chemical symbol Sm, specific gravity 2.60, atomic weight 87.8 (strontium).

Strontium is a metallic element whose properties resemble those of calcium. It is found in the earth and in spring water. Strontium salts are used for fireworks (they produce a red fire).

Nuclear experiments around the world caused the spread of the radioactive substance, strontium-90, and scientists claim that every human being has already absorbed quantities of it.

This dangerous radioactive substance accumulates in bones during the person's lifetime, and operates like X-rays in the body.

Strontium-90 has the following signs of toxicity: anemia and leukemia, bone cancer, and other forms of cancer.

You can protect yourself against toxicity by consuming the following: algin (from seaweed), and seaweed, pectin, which binds to the toxins in the intestines and prevents them from being absorbed, calcium and magnesium, yogurt and other fermented dairy products, vitamin B complex, lecithin, and the anti-oxidant vitamins.

Sulfur

Chemical symbol S, specific gravity 7, atomic weight 32 (sulphur).

Sulfur is a non-metallic element that is light orange in color, solid, brittle and soft, and highly flammable.

Sulfur is widespread in nature, and among other things it is used in pesticides and black gunpowder. Sulfur is also a component of a powerful acid called sulfuric acid, which is used in the petroleum industry, chemical waste, and dyestuffs.

Sulfur is linked to the consumption of protein, so that neglecting protein consumption (such as by not observing the basic law of food combinations) will cause a problem.

Sulfur is called the "beauty mineral" (despite its attendant odor, especially at sulfur spas), and it is therefore very important not to impair its absorption, since it also helps the blood to be more resistant to bacteria and infections. Moreover, it is found in keratin - the protein of the hair and nails, and in insulin.

Sulfur works with vitamin B complex to balance metabolism. In addition, it is important for the health of the hair, skin, and nails. It helps to balance the oxygen requirements and the activity of the brain. It assists the liver in the production of gall, and as a result, in breaking down fats. Sulfur combats bacterial infections,

Minerals

and is a component of amino acids: cystine, cysteine, methionine, and taurine, which are strong anti-oxidants and protect against toxicity. Experiments have shown that cysteine counteracts the toxicity of smoke and cigarette smoke.

Sulfur is also a component of biotin and thiamin (vitamin B1), which belong to the vitamin B group.

There is no daily recommended dietary allowance for sulfur. However, it is necessary to maintain the level and quality of proteins in the diet, so that sulfur can be absorbed effectively from the food.

Sulfur can be found in dried beans, fish, eggs, nuts (brazil nuts), lean meat, cabbage, Brussels sprouts, garlic, and onions.

If there is a shortage of sulfur, there is a possibility of hair, skin, or nail problems, and an increase in the body's difficulty to recover from toxicity. However, there are no known diseases resulting from a sulfur shortage.

Sulfur is not known to have toxic properties. The consumption of non-organic sulfur should be avoided.

Tin

Chemical symbol Sn, specific gravity 7.3, atomic weight 118.7 (stannum).

This is a white metal, silver in color, which the body requires for growth.

Little is known about the mechanisms at work in this mineral, except that its toxicity is harmful (like that of lead).

Traces of tin as a trace mineral are found both in plants and animals, and nothing is known about shortage or diseases caused by a shortage in the body.

Vanadium

Chemical symbol V, specific gravity 5.6, atomic weight 50.95 (vanadis).

Vanadium is a rare metal, white in color and similar to silver, which is used in the steel industry and for solidifying in the paint industry. This trace mineral is important for the human body, and even though all the body's requirements of this mineral are not yet known, researchers have found that it is linked to coronary heart diseases.

Vanadium is important for normal growth, as well as for the cholesterol in the body.

It is found in marine fish (abundantly), sea food, herrings, and sardines.

Signs of a shortage of vanadium are fairly rare, and are found in coronary heart diseases, growth, and cholesterol.

There is no toxicity in vanadium (unless synthetic vanadium is taken).

Zinc

Chemical symbol Zn, specific gravity 7.1, atomic weight 65.38 (zincum).

Zinc is a chemical element that belongs to the group of heavy metals.

It acts as a "traffic policeman" for the body's processes and enzyme maintenance.

The quantity of zinc in the body is the second highest of all the minerals, and it is of supreme importance, since it participates in the activities of over 70 enzymes in the digestive and metabolic systems.

Zinc is important for the functioning of the prostate gland and testes, and for the immune system; it helps heal wounds, and alleviates pain.

It is important to know that taking an increased quantity of zinc means that copper and vitamin B6 must also be taken, and it must be remembered that when there is a shortage of zinc, the immediate solution lies only in supplements, since it is difficult to compensate for shortages of zinc, or a demand for zinc, by means of food only.

Zinc is important in maintaining the acid-base balance in the body. It is one of the components of insulin - and for this reason, it is important for the body's sugar system. Moreover, it helps to release vitamin A from the liver, in this way benefiting vision. Zinc is essential for protein synthesis, as well as for the absorption and functioning of vitamins (especially from the B group). It is active in the immune system, kills bacteria, and fights cell degeneration, mainly with vitamins A, C, and selenium. For that reason, it is important in treating the mental deterioration that occurs as a result of Alzheimer's disease. It is important for brain activity and in the treatment of schizophrenia.

Zinc is an important component of the prostate gland, and is a component of seminal fluid. It is an important component in the menstrual cycle, in building the ovum, in sterility, and for sexual development in young people. It is important in the link between the hormonal system and the skin, such as acne problems. Zinc is essential for the skin; it is one of its components, and together with vitamins A, C, and E, treats severe skin problems.

Together with vitamins C and D, it is linked to the building of bones as the "cement" that joins calcium, magnesium and phosphorus. A link has been found to the curing of joint inflammation problems (together with other minerals).

Zinc is used to combat body odor, and, together with vitamin B6, serves as a natural deodorant. In addition, there is a link between zinc (+ vitamins B6 and A) and the senses of taste and smell. It helps to lower the cholesterol level.

The recommended daily amounts for infants of up to 6 months is 3 mg, for infants of between 6 and 12 months is 5 mg, for children of up to 10 years is 10 mg, and for people of 11 years and over is 15 mg. Pregnant women should take 20 mg, and nursing women should take 25 mg.

Children and adults with sugar problems or children who take vitamin B6 require more zinc, as do adults with prostate problems or who are undergoing treatment for problems such as impotence, aging (with manganese) and so on.

It should be remembered that zinc should be taken in conjunction with vitamins A, B6, calcium, and phosphorus. The best forms are chealated zinc, zinc gluconate, or zinc sulfate.

The foodstuffs that contain zinc are as follows: wheatgerm, bran, whole-wheat flour (whole-wheat bread), brown rice, sesame seeds, pumpkin seeds, most dried herbs, cashew nuts, nuts, almonds, eggs, legumes, and in smaller quantities in most vegetables.

When there is a shortage of zinc, the following symptoms can occur: prostate problems, especially enlargement of the gland (not a tumor). Many men ignore the fact that they are getting up more frequently at night, or run to the bathroom more often during the day, and this is a sign of prostate problems. Other symptoms are the slow healing of wounds and cuts, arteriosclerosis - hardening of the arteries, susceptibility to infections, increased fatigue and/or a loss of appetite, diabetic problems, white marks or spots on the nails, a loss of sensitivity to the taste and/or smell of food, and skin diseases (sometimes called "chronic").

While there is no toxicity in zinc, children

Minerals

should not take more than the recommended amounts (unless otherwise directed by a physician), because larger doses over time are liable to cause a shortage of copper, which can result in anemia or impaired heart rate/pulse. Adults should also not exceed the recommended amounts (unless otherwise directed by a physician). Remember to take the supplements.

Minerals

Astrolog Publishing House
P. O. Box 1123, Hod Hasharon 45111, Israel
Tel: 972-9-7412044
Fax: 972-9-7442714
E-Mail: info@astrolog.co.il
Astrolog Web Site: www.astrolog.co.il

Copyright © Jon Tillman 2000

ISBN 965-494-115-5

All rights reserved. No part of this publication may
be reproduced, stored in a retrieval system, or
transmitted, in any form or by any means, electronic,
mechanical, photocopying, recording or otherwise,
without the prior permission of the publisher.

Published by Astrolog Publishing House 2000

Printed in Israel
2 4 6 8 10 9 7 5 3 1